THE PROFESSIONAL RESIDENT SERVICE COORDINATOR

"Success is within reach"

Gregory Ford

INTRODUCTION:

Although, every employee is important to the operation of a housing community, the Resident Service Coordinator is the lifeline of a healthy, active and progressive community. Resident Service Coordinators serve as the liaison between management and residents. When it comes to advocating for enhancing the quality of life for residents, do it uniquely and do it correctly. In this book, you will find useful information on program development and on building a connected and engaged community. Resident Service Coordinators function best when they operate from a perspective of delivering service, building dignity in a person, and communicating the importance of human relationships. I found that being flexible, investigating conflicts objectively, using problem-solving skills and employing community-building strategies have allowed me to experience positive experiences within my community.

For me, defining the moment is about making the most of the time and position we have as Resident Service Coordinators. We should consistently look to empower residents, moving them to a state of greater independence. For example, when assisting residents who can't read to use bill pay services or with explaining the content of mail, take this opportunity to enroll the resident into a literacy program or a money management system. Simply doing activities of daily living on behalf of the resident stifles their growth and makes seniors or the disabled more accepting of and dependent upon institutionalization. As an RSC in Virginia, I defined my moment by assessing my community's needs, its strengths and relationships that I could build upon to address its requisite needs

Our position and time on earth is a gift that comes with a purpose: to live out our destiny and to help residents do the same. Time is not something that we can get back, nor do we know how much remains. People everywhere around the globe are constantly in search of more time to complete their responsibilities. Many complain that they never have enough time to live out their dreams. Therefore, it is important for RSCs to help residents maximize their time through achieving individual goals. This is why lifelong learning is so important. It communicates to that senior citizen or that disabled person or the single mother that life isn't over; there is always time to achieve a new goal. This approach has provided my residents the hope to obtain their GED as a grandmother, to become proficient in using a computer while having a learning disability, to repair their credit, to reconnect with family members, to start a savings account and to learn a new language.

Goal setting extends to you as the RSC as well. My goal is to incorporate individualized career planning and college preparation into affordable housing communities. The skill set of career planning and college prep strengthens the professional service of RSCs because it provides them with the tools to deliver a much-needed service in affordable housing family communities.

Resident Service Coordinators are vital to identifying resident issues and needs and are vital to helping to mitigate those situations. One role of the RSC (Resident Service Coordinator) is to identify resources and to link residents to those resources. The RSC facilitates weekly educational programs with the goal of enhancing residents' quality of life. Since RSCs serve as the primary contact for residents, earning the resident's trust is important. Start by working to differentiate your services from the services offered outside of your community for the goal of the RSC program is to avoid the duplication of existing community-based services. Communicate both verbally and non-verbally that you are specifically working to advance your specific community and that you have a personal stake in the happiness and well-being of your residents.

I found that being organized, offering reassurance, being flexible and operating under transparency wins residents trust.

Organizations begin with having file systems that are easily accessible, secured and filled with current information. There's simply nothing worse for a resident than experiencing a conversation with a worker who has misplaced paperwork, and is clearly unprepared to address the resident's concerns. I found it most effective to be upfront and forthright at the outset of completing an intake assessment of a resident or when addressing resident concerns. Provide follow up with residents to demonstrate that you have completed agreed upon tasks. Residents will appreciate the individual attention and effort that you put into their concerns. Residents want to hear that not only you have helped them achieve their goals but how and when. Therefore, it's only natural that residents will feel the need to be reassured that their matters have been resolved.

Your number one goal for your first meeting with a resident is to get a clear picture of the resident's life situation and to look for ways that you can contribute. Use good listening skills; make it less about you and more about the resident. This builds trust. Most residents hold back until they believe that the RSC is there to help them. The quality of the intake assessment determines your future relationship with a resident. Let residents know that you've listened to them, that you understand them and that you most definitely will work to help them. Working with residents does pose some challenges, so not only is good relationship building needed but also good program development skills.

Chapter 1: Conflict in the House

Conflict amongst residents as well as residents and staff can be disruptive to the atmosphere of the community; but it is an opportunity to do your thing! Bringing people together from various backgrounds and various life experiences to live under one roof is bound to bring conflict. Conflicts can range from racial intolerances to ideological differences. Seize the opportunity to help your residents by defining the moment. Programs that address resident conflict include:

I.   Solving differences by creating a debate team

This is a great way to educate your residents. The debate requires researching information, articulating your thoughts in a convincing manner, respecting the beliefs of others, acknowledging the facts and discarding rumors or personal experience.[1] The benefits are:

- helping residents to develop self-awareness,

- improving listening skills, and enhancing concentration skills,

- improving people skills

---

[1] Idebate.org

- helping residents to become smarter,

- allow for cultural exchange and

- to build greater community awareness.

II. Empower residents by helping them to facilitate a staff-training workshop.

Developing an effective staff-training program is vital to the long-term success of any business. Training programs provide multiple benefits for employees and the community, but only if they are carefully planned and properly implemented. Training is a means to a specific end, so keeping goals in mind during the development and implementation stages of your training program will assist in creating a clearly defined and effective program.

Resident sponsored staff training allows residents a venue to communicate the importance of treating them with dignity and the understanding of what is it like to be a resident in an affordable housing community. The preparation for the workshop should involve tasks that engage the residents in self-assessment exercises and include activities on promoting effective dialogue with staff. Residents are more inclined to change their negative behavior when they recognize a more viable option for interacting with others. This back door approach is very effective.

If you like the ideal of a staff training, start with a survey to identify the issues and concerns that you wish to address in the training. The success of data collection requires careful preparation. The first and often the most difficult question is "Why am I doing this survey?"

The Four Main Reasons to Conduct Surveys

Susan E. Wyse on June 29, 2012

RSCs should embrace the business approach by conducting surveys to uncover answers to specific, important questions. These questions are varied, cover a diverse range of topics, and can be asked in multiple formats. When structuring your survey questions, consider the following:

What are the four main reasons why businesses and researchers should conduct surveys?

1. To uncover the answers - In a non-intimidating survey environment, you will learn about what motivates residents and what is important to them, and gather meaningful opinions, comments, and feedback. A non-intimidating survey environment is one that best suits the privacy needs

of the resident. Respondents are more likely to provide open and honest feedback in a more private survey method. Methods such as online surveys, paper surveys, or mobile surveys are more private and less intimidating than face-to-face survey interviews or telephone surveys.

2. To evoke discussion - Give your survey respondents an opportunity to discuss important key topics. Communicate with your respondents about your survey topic. This allows you to dig deeper into your survey, and can incite topics related to your survey within a broader perspective.

3. To base decisions on objective information - Conducting surveys is an unbiased approach to decision-making. You can collect unbiased survey data and develop sensible decisions based on analyzed results. By analyzing results, you can immediately address topics of importance, rather than waste time and valuable resources on areas of little or no concern.

4. To compare results - Surveys results provide a snapshot of the attitudes and behaviors – including thoughts, opinions, and comments – about your target survey population. This valuable feedback is your baseline to measure and establish a benchmark from which to compare results over time

III. Create a Resident Action Committee (RAC).

The RAC is bringing residents together to discuss ways to collectively improve the community. It starts by identifying issues that strongly concern the majority of the residents. Coordinate the conversation so it stays focused on one particular agreed upon issue. The task is to generate energy so that the residents can develop solution-focused suggestions for resolving resident/community based concerns. When residents come together with the opportunity to apply their vision, values, life experiences and knowledge towards advancing the agenda, a healthy community should result. The solution-focused approach targets the desired outcome established at the resident action committee meetings. This is a great tool for producing solutions and avoiding complaining sessions about the community or speaking poorly of staff. At the start of my monthly RAC meetings, I start by reminding residents that our discussions provide them with the opportunity to influence community policies and thus meetings must stay on topic and be positive in our approach.

Chapter 2: Help Residents With The Transition To Your Community

Roll out the "red carpet." Make new residents feel proud, and honored to be a member of their community by highlighting its many positive attributes. Your community might not be a four or five star resort but it has many positive attributes and positive people within it, and this should be emphasized. When you roll out the red carpet, residents will view affordable housing as a right to all citizens and will feel privileged to live in their community. Then, new residents will be more likely to assume personal responsibility for the upkeep of the community. Residents will in turn challenge themselves to bring something positive to the community.

For example, the retired math teacher might lend her math skills to the RSC GED program, and the new resident who was once a cook might help other residents understand the benefits of consuming well-balanced meals. Every resident has something to contribute to the community, but first you must give them a reason to do so.

One way to achieve a culture where new residents become a meaningful part of the community and integrate smoothly is to use visual aids. Host a brunch and show video interviews of current residents who are the model residents: such residents are engaged, have a positive disposition, are goal oriented, approachable and care for their community. It could be one minute per person for a twelve-minute video. Ask open-ended questions such as

- Explain how this community has improved your life.

- In what ways have you contributed to the community?

- What should people know about living in affordable housing?

- What makes you smile?

- Give your definition or vision of a good community.

Questions like these draw people in and help new residents to imagine a place for themselves in their new community. After watching the video, new residents are likely to feel safer, more at ease, and more secure in their decision to move into your community.

RSCs conduct intake assessments of new residents with the best intentions; learning about the residents and their needs. However, in writing this book, I have come to realize that my intake assessments have had more misses than hits. Yes, it gathers the basic demographic information, such as emergency contacts, name of physician and consent forms. But asking other information such as the following would be extremely helpful:

1. List two things that you like to do in your free time.

2. List two strengths that you have.

3. List a weakness that you have that you would like to improve.

4. Name one person you would most want to be like.

5. Your favorite food is:

6. What do you usually do when you are lonely?

7. What do you usually do when you are angry?

8. You are happiest when:

9. Something that make me laugh is:

10. The best time of the day is:

11. Your most memorable moment is:

12. I think I am a good person because:

13. If I was the Resident of the Year, it would be because:

This type of conversation will provide the RSC a great perspective of the new residents. It allows the residents to reflect on his or her life and residents will be more inclined to search for ways to be happy and a part of the community. The goal of being Resident of the Year has just become a possibility!

Create a welcome packet that includes free admission to community programs. If you provide new residents with a personal invitation, they will be more likely to attend.

CHAPTER 3: LIVING WELL IS BEING HEALTHY

In an independent living community, residents are ultimately responsible for their own health and well-being. However, not helping residents to be healthy and safe is a failed business strategy. Healthy residents equal less turn over in the apartments, which translate to greater stability and greater profit for the business. Establish a resident monitoring program where one of the residents is assigned to check on the well-being of other community members. In turn, that resident hall monitor has someone to check on his or her well-being. Each resident would place a sign stating "I'm Okay today" on the front of his or her door by 10:00am every morning. This alerts the resident monitor that that individual is not in need of immediate medical attention. This is not a foolproof program but rather a small step towards helping a resident that may have experienced a medical emergency or injury while in his or her apartment. The Resident Service Coordinator should meet monthly with the hall monitors to address any concerns and to obtain an update on what is occurring in the community. Not only will hall monitors report on the well-being of residents assigned to them, but also hall monitors can report any increase of trash in the stairwells, people loitering, the concerns of other residents, noise complaints, etc. Residents tend to view the hall monitor as the person that they can confide in.

Host a town hall meeting and ask your residents if they would benefit from having a wellness clinic and if so, what medical needs would they like to see addressed. Some common health issues and needs that you will likely be addressing are blood pressure checks, diabetes screening, medication management, and mental health services. The wellness clinic can provide preventative health services. Pressured by an aging and increasingly complex population, healthcare delivery and healthcare professional education is undergoing change. Rising healthcare costs and marked variability in the intensity of care without corresponding improvements in population health suggest that there is great need for a wellness clinic in these communities. Often, populations with a higher burden of chronic illness and poorly coordinated care cluster in underserved healthcare settings that can benefit from targeted healthcare interventions. These common chronic illnesses often lead to greater medical complications. For example, diabetes can lead to:

•Heart Disease – People with diabetes have a higher risk for heart attack and stroke.

•Eye Complications – People with diabetes have a higher risk of blindness and other vision problems.

•Kidney Disease – Diabetes can damage the kidneys and may lead to kidney failure with the need for dialysis.

•Nerve Damage (neuropathy) – Diabetes can cause damage to the nerves that run through the body.

•Foot Problems – Nerve damage, infections of the feet, and problems with blood flow to the feet can be caused by diabetes.

•Skin Complications – Diabetes can cause skin problems, such as infections, sores, and itching. Skin problems are sometimes a first sign that someone has diabetes.

•Dental Disease – Diabetes can lead to problems with teeth and gums, called gingivitis and periodontitis.

HTN hypertension and diabetes frequently cause renal compromise and/or renal failure.

Your kidneys filter excess fluid and waste from your blood, a process that depends on healthy blood vessels. High blood pressure can injure both the blood vessels in and leading to your kidneys, causing several types of kidney disease (nephropathy). Having diabetes in addition to high blood pressure can worsen the damage. High blood pressure (hypertension) can quietly damage your body for years before symptoms develop. Left uncontrolled, you may wind up with a disability, a poor quality of life or even a fatal heart attack. This is why preventive care is so important. Health issues can be addressed before they become major issues.[2]

Link pharmacy delivery service to your wellness clinic. Having medications delivered to the home of the residents reduces the chances of days of not taking medication because of barriers to getting to the pharmacy. In addition, having medications delivered to the residential site allows for medication management by the wellness clinic pharmacist, allows for free bubble wrap packaging of the medications, flu shot and other vaccination services at home.

Having residents who are sexually active is very common. It doesn't matter if your residents are over 62, with a disability, or religious and under the age of 21, sex education is a health service that should be provided. People of all ages usually derive information on sex and related subjects from sources such as friends, books, media advertising, soap operas and reality shows, television, magazines and the Internet. The

---

[2] www.webmd.com

problem is that these sources may or may not provide them with accurate information. As such, sex education will help in communicating authentic information and in the process correct any misinformation that may have been embraced. No one wants to think about grandma and/or grandpa having sex. But the truth of the matter is that some older people are still interested in engaging in sex and are sexually active. Roughly 53% of people aged 65 to 74 are sexually active and 26% of people aged 75 to 85 are engaged in sexual activity. It is important to note that sex education consists of more than using protection when having intercourse.

For older adults, sex is not as simple as finding a partner, arming oneself with protection and engaging in a consensual and enjoyable experience. As we age, being sexually active becomes more challenging. In general, we face a number of health and physical issues that limit our capacity to engage in sex safely. Certain age-related ailments such as arthritis, heart conditions, loss of collagen decreasing one's flexibility and others impact the body's ability to fully enjoy intercourse. Another aspect of senior sexuality that is even more rarely discussed is that of sexually transmitted infections, also known as STIs. One study recently found that the prevalence of genital herpes among individuals age 70 and older was 28% with the percentage being still higher among women. An additional concern to be aware of is that for women, some STIs can replicate or have similar symptoms to certain aspects of menopause. The presence of HIV (Human Immunodeficiency Virus) has recently been increasing among older adults with about 10% of new HIV cases in the U.S. being diagnosed among seniors. Safe sex education is provided to teens in high school, however little to no education and outreach is provided for older adults, even though they are a high-risk population for acquiring the disease. Some sexually active seniors feel that since they are no longer able to reproduce, they cannot get an STI and do not need to use a condom. This huge misconception has unfortunately affected many seniors. The Center for Disease Control projects that by 2015, half of all individuals who have HIV in our country will be seniors and more than one third of them will be women. These startling statistics reinforce the significant need for better education and outreach to sexually active senior members of our communities. Make learning fun to fully engage the audience and help them walkaway with a take home message. One recommended activity is using starburst candy: Residents of an age 55 or 62 and older community are more likely to experience larger incidences of hospitalization than traditional communities.

A homebound program allows the Resident Service Coordinator to work with hospitals, social workers, family members, residents and the discharge planner to coordinate a safe transition back to the community following hospitalization. RSCs are knowledgeable of the environment to which the residents are returning thus are in a position to help clinically, socially and psychologically to give insight on resources that can help the residents return to an independent functioning state. In addition, the bond between residents who are hospitalized, their family members and RSCs strengthens when RSCs serve in an advocacy capacity. Avoid steering the resident to particular companies that provide home health services, medical equipment or a particular pharmacist. Always allow the resident the option to select the service provider with whom he or she is most comfortable.

The future of smoking:

Many businesses have gone smoke-free and many more businesses will likely follow. Even housing communities are considering the benefits of being a smoke-free community. Be ahead of the curve in the event that your community goes smoke-free by offering smoking cessation classes. In addition to health benefits, there is an economic windfall for residents who reduce the use of cigarettes or quit altogether. It's never too late to stop smoking. Seniors of any age can reap many benefits from quitting smoking and improve their overall health as well as add years to their lives. Many smokers experience a range of health problems from lung disease to cancer. Everyday life can be drastically improved simply by stopping smoking. If you are a senior who smokes, consider the many benefits that *you* can experience if you quit the habit. Quitting now, will give you a longer life and will decrease your chances of having a disease associated with smoking.

Resources to Help You Establish Smoking Cessation Programs:

•NCI (National Cancer Institute) Smoking Quit line: Call the Quit line at 1-877-44U-QUIT to get personal counseling as well as printed materials to help you quit smoking.

•Smokefree.gov: Created by the NCI, this site features a step-by-step guide to quitting as well as resources such as online quizzes, tools that can help you quit and guides to medications as well as links to resources in your area.

•American Cancer Society: The ACS offers The Guide to Quitting Smoking as well as brochures on preventing and treating cancer. To order free materials by phone, call 1-800-227-2345. If you have a friend or family member who smokes, ask them to quit along with you. The more support you have, the easier the process will be. Friends and family know you best, and can help you through the tough times and encourage you to quit the habit of smoking to improve your health.

The pharmacist from your wellness clinic is a great resource for running a smoking cessation program. I was fortunate to work with the pharmacist from Virginia Commonwealth University School of Pharmacy in developing a stop smoking program for our community. The class met weekly for two hours. The program started with 12 residents and quickly grew to 15. Residents were excited and eager to take the step to stop smoking or reduce the amount of cigarettes they consumed. The smoking cessation program's name was changed to smoking class to reduce the stigma at the request of the residents. The smoking class included a pharmacist intern, pharmacist and resident service coordinator.

After 6 weeks of smoking classes, the following findings were noted:

Significant challenges emerged in attempting to curb the smoking habits of people who had been smoking for more than 30 years, were low income and who had numerous health conditions:

1. Fear of losing friendship.
    a. As residents committed reducing or eliminating the use of cigarettes, they expressed concern over how their

       participation in a smoking class would affect their friendship with family members, peers, and friends who smoked.

   b. One solution to this issue is to use social work interns to coach the residents and help them to recognize the value of personal growth and improved individual health.

2. Fear of weight gain.

   a. There was a lot of misinformation and rumors that residents cling to as justification for why they can't quit smoking

   b. Solution would be to encourage residents to participate in the community's programs such as the eating smart, exercise, and the wellness clinic. Encourage residents to work with their primary care physician on establishing a weight loss program.

3. Hope of a quick solution

   a. Residents had an expectation of immediate results, especially when residents learned that their cohorts were making significant strides in reducing their cigarette use.

   b. Our solution was to operate under a hybrid approach. This consists of group and individual smoking counseling sessions. The goal is show residents how one strategy doesn't necessarily work for all and that participating in group and individual smoking sessions is important. RSC are in place to help the residents move from positions of shame, embarrassment, and hopelessness to one of strength and triumph. Under the hybrid system, we would have weekly topics such as:

    i. Finances (the fiscal cost of cigarettes annually)

    ii. Characteristics of a smoker and which methods and agents best accommodate certain individuals

    iii. Goal setting - one size doesn't fit all

    iv. Behavior clues for relapsing (trigger to smoke)

c. There is a need for behavioral modification and motivational interviewing to keep a resident engaged.

4. No one cares about me.

a. Residents are generally aware that smoking has harmful effects but slip into the belief that no one cares about their health anyway. Residents struggled with not being able to report positive news while others were reporting gains from attending the class. For residents who did not make progress, the smoking class was seen as punitive.

b. The solution is to launch a quit smoking campaign that includes verbiage and visual aids that you care and support them. Utilize guest speakers so that residents can hear the quit smoking message from others. A budget for guest speakers is recommended. Offer prizes for 1 month, 2 months and 3 months of perfect attendance to incentivize the residents to stick with the program. Offer healthy snacks during the meetings to help residents focus on the subject matter.

5. Low literacy
    a. Many of our residents read on a level that is less than proficient to read the literature assimilated pertaining to smoking. Especially smoking related medical literature
    b. The solution is to provide reading material at the 5th grade level.
6. Fluctuation in attendance
    a. Residents would join the meeting weeks into the session. This created some disruption to the flow of the meetings.
    b. The solution was to operate future meetings under a closed ended form with a registration period that closes at the start of the class. New residents could join future sessions once sign up reached six residents.

7. Health status

    a. It is essential to know the medical condition of the residents because residents would be using nicotine replacement agents such as "The Patch," Nicotine Gum, prescribed medications, etc. Some residents do not have a physician and the question of who will monitor the resident's usage of nicotine replacement without a physician creates risks.

    b. The solution is to establish a working relationship with the primary care provider; establish a Memorandum of Understanding (M.O.U.) affiliation agreement. Under the agreement, physicians would prescribe replacement therapy and the smoking class would serve as the eyes and ears on the ground and co-managing nicotine replacement therapy because out of pocket cost would be a deterrent to resident obtaining medication.

8. The smoking class would like to budget for a stipend for two interns: one social work student and one pharmacy student. Keeping residents motivated is vital to the success of the class.

Establish a transportation service for residents to reduce barriers to keeping medical appointments. One efficient transportation program is Dr. Transportation, which transports residents within a senior or persons with disability housing community to medical appointments twice a month for $2.00 round trip. Residents are provided the dates that transportation will be available one month in advance which allows residents to schedule medical appointments for those dates.

Chapter 4: Continuous Learning

Lifelong learning is the minimum requirement for self-fulfillment and personal achievement. The institutions, organizations and resources that our residents depend on operate in the 21st century. Our residents would be better consumers if they function as a 21st century people.

This brings us to a very important point on intelligence, information, and lifelong learning. There are several different kinds of education that your residents can acquire, either deliberately or in a random, haphazard fashion. Two of these kinds of learning are maintenance learning, and growth learning. Maintenance learning refers to your keeping current with the things around you such as reading about gains being made in medical technology or policies being debated in a presidential election.

Maintenance learning is essential. It is very similar to the light physical exercise that keeps you at a particular level of fitness that keeps you somewhat healthy.

The second type of learning is growth learning. This is the kind of learning that adds knowledge and skills to the resident's repertoire of learning that they did not have before. For example, if a resident decides to learn to speak Spanish so that he or she can expand their opportunities to work or volunteer in the Hispanic community, every word, phrase and sentence that he or she learns is a form of growth learning. Growth learning helps residents expand their mind and acquire information that they did not have before and enables them to do things that they could not do before. RSCs can establish programs that promote continuous learning. Some suggestions include:

Literacy programs, which help residents to communicate better with their medical providers, read their mail, understand conversation with others, understand the world around them better, pursue dreams and aspirations and feel better about themselves. A RSC should link up with the public school system to offer GED classes, computer training classes, and free college courses for senior citizens.

People respond well to an entertaining program, especially one with incentives. A great incentive for learning and reading is to establish a Book Club.

Good Health Includes Reading:

Book Club

Objective: to improve the reading skills of residents; to influence the conservation conversation of residents to take on more positive discussions in common areas; to help residents understand the health benefits of literacy and education; to expand the resident's knowledge base.

Format:

• Closed ended monthly sessions (once the Book Club has begun reading the selected book, new members can't join until the club has completed reading the book).

• Members meet weekly in the library.

• Members must begin participation in the Book Club at the beginning of each month, as participation will not be permitted once members have begun reading the selected book. New members can join the book club prior to the start of the new book.

• Meetings will include reading the book aloud, mini quizzes on the book's content, and discussion of the book.

- Mini quizzes and group discussions will be used to verify that residents are reading on pace and understanding the content of the book.

- Residents will be assigned to read certain book chapters between classes and should be prepared to discuss what they read.

- Guest speakers will be used occasionally as it relates to the subject matter.

- Supplemental items will be introduced at meetings to help residents better identify with the subject matter. For example, the book *Slum Dog Millionaire* covers the India/Asia culture and class system. Thus, readers would be introduced to Indian cuisine that was likely consumed by the subjects in the book. In addition, a guest speaker would likely be a person of the Indian culture who could expand on the book teachings.

- Connected Living - Connected Living is a computer based program service that combines technology, programming and people. Connected Living supports computer instructors with the tasks of engaging residents with computer operations into their daily lives. I was able to have Connected Living program in conjunction with the Book of the

Month, and capture quotes from residents on their thoughts and impressions of the book.

- Upon completion of reading the assigned book, residents will work with Connected Living Ambassador to produce a one-page book report as follows:

  - Describe the content of the book

  - What impact did the book have on your life?

- RSC will apply for the approval of deducting $10 from the resident's rent upon the completion of reading the assigned book and submitting an approved one-page book report created using Connected Living. The Book Club will be evaluated quarterly to ensure that the target goals are being met.

There are clear benefits to having positive relationships with others. The book club can achieve this while meeting other needs of the residents. For some residents, the book club represents time away from their daily routine; others like to learn new things and some cherish the friendships developed within the group. Having a network of friends can boost our immune systems and be a buffer to stress (Robert Putnam, Bowling Alone: New York: Simon & Schuster, 2000). With friends and book club associates, we are happier, less depressed, have higher self-esteem, and are more skilled and prosperous. Those with relationships tend to live longer and a book club is a great way to have a fuller life.

CHAPTER 5: WHAT IS THE DEAL WITH THE MONEY?

Living on a fixed income can present many challenges for seniors, single parents and persons with disabilities. The ability to earn additional income is very limited and often non-existent. It is important that Resident Service Coordinators help residents develop a plan to spend their money wisely.

Establish a couponing program that teaches residents how to use the computer to clip coupons for daily grocery shopping and help stretch their income. Place a coupon exchange box in a common area where residents can take coupons and place coupons in return. Couponing can not only save the residents money, but it also psychologically shifts their mindset to being aware of how they spend money. Having quarterly meetings with residents to discuss the effectiveness of the couponing program is essential. Program review allows feedback on the program and provides residents a role in discussing ways to build on the program. Quarterly meetings with the coupon program participants is a great opportunity to host workshops on how to establish a saving plan; education on the price mark-ups on products and goods at convenient stores versus traditional grocery store chains; how eating healthy can be affordable, and daily money management.

Do not be judgmental however do educate your residents how low income people have a tendency to buy expensive clothes and accessories that exceeds their means. Capitalism is powerful in convincing those who cannot afford it that they need highly fashionable shoes, purses and clothes. When we watch a lot of television, listen to radio and search the web, we become the targets of advertisement. What this creates is an image of products that people believe they must have; should I Jordans? Basketball players believe that having a pair will make them jump higher and students believe that will be "cooler" and more accepted by their peers, if they get some Jordans. You can have the conversation of how a pair of Jordans cost Nike $10 to produce but can cost the as much as $186. I have observed residents who are on a fixed income become stressed trying to acquire money to purchase their kids and grandkids trendy sneakers. A pair of Jordans could offer a breakthrough discussion on money management, leading your residents into financial stability.

Many of my own residents would scoff at the idea of applying for food stamps because they feel that very little could be purchased for $15 a month. Incorporating the use of couponing along with smart shopping strategies can greatly expand residents' buying power. Do not hesitate to approach grocery stores managers and regional managers to set up shopping education seminars for your residents. Managers can share marketing strategies, pricing tactics, sale trends, understanding nutritional values and the difference between brand name and generic brand foods. Managers are open to educating consumers because informed consumers are loyal and happy consumers. Companies spend a lot of money on advertising to get consumers to buy their brand. In most instances, the store brand or generic brand costs less and usually tastes the same. In fact, they often use the very same ingredient. Host a blind taste test of products with residents at the coupon meeting to illustrate how residents can have the same taste for less. Again, you are empowering residents to make wise choices. In the end, the company that makes the brand name often also makes the generic brand. Some generic brands will be more favorable than others so try and then decide.

Welcome to the 21st Century:

Introduce your residents to online banking and online rent payment as a way of saving time, money and gaining peace of mind. Residents who aren't computer savvy might be reluctant to embrace electronic monetary transactions. Facilitate educational workshops on the benefits to residents of electronic bill pay. Your property will see increased number of signed leases, improved collection rates, improved occupancy rates by allowing prospective residents to pay their security deposits electronically.

As a Resident Service Coordinator, I had residents who were on fixed incomes carrying cash to convenient stores to purchase money orders to pay their rent. This places them in position to be robbed and costs them annually $24.00 in money order purchases. The $24.00 in annual saving can be applied to the resident's grocery shopping expense account, meeting their nutritional needs. In addition, when residents are hospitalized they become increasingly worried about getting out of the hospital to cash their social security express debit cards. The stress of worrying about paying rent on time when hospitalized creates stress and can cause further decline in health. Knowing that your rent is paid in full and on time is peaceful and reassuring.

CHAPTER 6: EMPLOYMENT

Too often, people view communities where residents are over 62 or disabled as a place where people stop growing. With this thinking, we lose tons of knowledge and skills that these residents could add to the workforce. There is actual value in life experience, work experience and withstanding the test of time. In 2010, 6.6 million people over age 65 worked or looked for work in the first six months of the year. That analysis is based on federal records. As Resident Service Coordinator, it is likely that many of your residents will be interested in acquiring part-time employment, maintaining their employment or with developing the skills necessary to enter the workforce. Working can be self-fulfilling as it contributes to the value of life. Working also includes volunteer service as well. I strongly recommend program development to address this need.

Establish partnerships with organizations such as Catholic Charities, Urban League, Senior Connections, and AmeriCorps for assistance with identifying job opportunities for persons over 62 and/or with disabilities.

Career planning and job retention can be met through a job-training workshop. The workshop would run for six days straight bi-annually.

Programming can be a great way to bring out the fundamental dignity of each resident. RSCs should commit to helping provide that opportunity, especially to the most vulnerable and marginalized populations.

CHAPTER 7: ENGAGE AND COMMUNICATE

Resident Service Coordinators — whether you know it or not, you are at the brink of your defining moment. You are putting in countless hours so that you can experience the joy a much-deserved progressive community. You are consistently developing your skills and knowledge to make sure that you have the endurance and ability to complete the task. You are making a courageous attempt to be all that you can be so that you can one day be considered a legendary RSC. The key is to understand that inviting, healthy and well manicured communities are not just limited to market rate communities. You may have hopes and dreams of having a model, four star community thus you need a campaign to communicate your vision and ambassadors that live within the community to share this vision. Preparation to achieve success in transforming a community is extremely commendable, so let's begin.

A quality monthly newsletter sets the tone of the community, influences the culture and communicates the services and programs that are available to residents. If you desire an active community, produce an active newsletter. Newsletters are also a great way to keep in touch with current residents. You can provide an even broader audience (families, community members, visitors) with helpful information and tips and announcing upcoming events and activities.

Have an open communication with your customers, stockholders and employees. You are the one who knows your service the best, and by communicating directly with your residents and employees, you show them you care about them, too. You can give detailed explanations on policies and introduce strategies to improve the quality of life for residents and employees. Newsletters allow residents the opportunity to share their experiences of living within the community.

Family forum is a great tool for celebrating your residents while strengthening their support systems from family members and friends. As a RSC, I hosted a family forum by distributing invitations to residents and their love ones. The forum features the residents as the panel of experts and the family as the audience. Below is how the family forum was rolled out:

"Hello and thank you all for attending our first Family Forum. Today's goal is to celebrate you and your loved ones. As an RSC, I follow the lead of my wonderful supervisors (Tom Stokes and Brenda Limone) and operate under the vision of Beacon Communities LLC. Beacon believes in affordable housing and that every individual should have access to quality housing within a healthy environment.

My name is Gregory Ford and I am the Resident Service Coordinator (RSC). My primary role is to work beside the residents to improve their quality of life and to assist residents in achieving their life goals or to age in place gracefully.

Three years ago, I walked into the doors of my current employer eager to work with seniors and become a part of the community. My first introduction to the culture came when a resident gave me some advice:

1.   Don't judge us!

2.   Don't underestimate us!

3.   Stay out of my way!

This was my introduction that my seniors are very different from the nursing home clients that I had served for eight years. So, three years later, I have learned not to judge my residents, I don't underestimate my resident's will or abilities and I am learning to stay out of the way of Ms. James.

Programs that I along with partners from the community have incorporated into the community include:

- Mammogram screening

- Youth mentoring program

- Spanish class

- Pet owners' club

In surveying the community, it became apparent that the twenty residents who had pets were very compassionate about being pet owners. I worked to capture this energy and love for animals by bringing residents together to share the role of pet ownership with others. I hosted monthly meetings with various speakers from the pet community. Workshops for the pet owners included: how yoga for dogs can relieve tension in pets and their owner, best practices for caring for cats and dogs in a high rise building within an urban setting, bereavement resources during the loss of a pet, meals on wheels nutrition assistance for dogs and cats, and veterinary care. I was able to establish a medical care program for the pets for which I contracted with a vet to conduct home visits to treat our animals. Management agreed to subsidize the vet care to ensure that our resident's pets were receiving the vaccinations, grooming and emergency care that was needed. Pets are like family to residents so keeping animals healthy helps keep residents healthy as well.

- Alcoholics Anonymous

It is most important that the Resident Service Coordinator understand the characteristics of the resident population and property you serve. Issues that may impact the differential use of services are socioeconomic, age, culture, gender, race, sexual orientation and others. There will be different expectations and concerns based on your location. A property in a community in rural Iowa has different issues than properties in inner city Richmond. For instance, when deciding whether to offer an Alcoholics Anonymous program, I had to assess whether our community would be overrun by persons in the surrounding area attending our Alcoholics Anonymous meetings. Because our community is in a high crime area, I had to develop an AA program center on safety and strict boundaries so residents could be protected. In response to high alcohol consumption and the increase of alcohol related issues, an Alcoholics Anonymous program was established within our building. We also recognized that a number of our residents were becoming dependent on the use of alcohol on a daily basis. My residents would smell like alcohol early in the morning, I witnessed increased arguments where alcohol was present; I saw the use of alcohol to cope with life issues and noticed that residents were increasingly exhibiting alcohol induced health related illnesses such as hand tremors, stomach problems and blackouts. And there were Incidents where residents were hallucinating and experiencing paranoia. So, I began an Alcoholics Anonymous program, I opened the meetings up to the community within a one mile radius and to traveling Alcoholics Anonymous members who may be on business travel and our site is the nearest meeting. In establishing RSC programs, it is beneficial to offer services that connect the community to your residents. Don't be a community that is only on the receiving end, be a community that gives back. To distinguish our community, we offered:

- CPR training

- Stop Smoking classes

- Diabetes Club

- The Wellness Clinic

- The Women's Club

- Connected Living

- Conflict Resolution workshops

- Financial Planning workshops

- Public Safety workshops

- Self-defense class

- Voter registration drive

- Voting rights restoration

- Bedbug Prevention workshop

- Town Hall meetings

- Elder Abuse workshops

- Health Fair

- Car Transfer safety

- Fall prevention and walker evaluations

- 12 week nutrition class

- $2.00 hair cuts

The Resident Service Coordinator program offers many benefits to the residents, management, housing owners, taxpayers and the local government. The following are some of the many advantages of the program such as, prevents hoarding, educates the staff on best practices for working with residents, elevates the self-esteem and independence of residents, strengthens management and independence of residents, enhances the value of the community and establishes a reduction in eviction rates and resident conflicts. The first six months of employment as a Resident Service Coordinator, I wanted to deliver a service that was beneficial to many residents while connecting a new RSC program to the community. I canvased the neighborhood becoming familiar with local businesses and the people who run them. I was able to convince the local barber to offer two-dollar haircuts every Monday from 9:00am – 12:00. My residents were given appointments and I would provide the barber with the list on the Friday prior. The regular haircut price at this barbershop was $14.00 and now our residents had access to professional haircut services for both men and women at an economical price. The barbershop was clean, wheelchair accessible and functioned within a positive environment. Positive environment referred to being respectful, and intellectually stimulating and witty conversation within the shop. The $2.00 haircut program unfortunately ended when a resident went rogue, and visited the barbershop outside the agreed upon appointment time and repeatedly interrupted the barbers' normal business operation.

What I learned from this experience is that I should have been proactive in emphasizing the importance of residents conforming to the barbershop policy agreement. I should have also informed residents how individual acts reflect on the whole community. The strength of desire to conform is a personality trait whereby some people will try to conform to whatever group they are in at the time, while other 'non-conformists' will go in the other direction, deliberately asserting their individuality by rejecting all but a very few set of norms.

So, if you want to persuade someone, it helps a great deal to gain their trust by being in the same group as them; highlighting that you are a part of their community. For example, a RSC may go down to a barbershop with the residents and get a haircut along with them.

I should have had an intervention plan in place in the event that residents showed up at the barbershop at non-appointment times. This would have prepared the barber for situations when residents were non-compliant.

- Tours of assisted living and nursing homes

- Yoga for Seniors

- Social work interns

- New tenant welcome committee

- Free dental care including dentures

- Understanding Medicare workshops

- Fraud Prevention and scams on seniors

- The Homebound Program

- An enhanced lunch program

- This Family Forum

- Sex Education

And yes, family, our residents have participated in three sex education classes. The classes seem to draw more folks every time. For some residents, sex education is a way to become more knowledgeable about the risks and health benefits associated with intimacy while others understand the importance of being able to have that all important conversation with their grandchildren. Remember, my role is to educate, provide resources and stay out of the way.

Future programs coming to our location include:

1. Sign language class

2. Safe driving course for seniors

3. GED - 12 week course

4. Literacy program

5. Mental health services

6. A Community Resident video

7.   Online rent payment

8.   Engaging, educating and building partnerships with the home health nurses and aides

9.   Partnership with local grocery store

10.   Art appreciation class for drawing, painting and sculpture

11.   Bremo Pharmacy services

Family Forum:

Too often, family members guess at what type of support their loved ones want, need or expect. The Family Forum is a good way to open up dialogue, share experiences, share thoughts and hopes of strengthening relationships, opening up dialogue and bringing our community closer together. So, instead of supporting Mom when she becomes ill, the forum shows the importance of supporting Mom while she is healthy, both physically and mentally. The local university gerontology professor served as the moderator and asked residents to answer the following questions in the presence of their love ones:

As you consider your role in life, please share what that role looks like ...

In what ways do you think your mom or dad is like you?

Who is the person who influenced your life the most?

What was the happiest moment of your life?

What are the most important lessons that you have learned in life?

What is your fondest memory of me?

When you were my age, what was your favorite thing to do?

As my parent, how would you like me to treat you?

How would you like to be remembered?

How can I make you smile?

What is the best thing that money can't buy that I can give you?

When I speak about you to my friends, I say the following: ___________________.

My dream vacation is ___________________________.

I do the following things in hopes that it will bring you good fortune: ___________________________________.

The time when I worry about you the most is ___________________.

Cooking for one person is___________________________.

What is life like at the age of _________________________?

As I grow older, I expect ________________ from my family.

~

Computer training courses to promote using Skype, and email:

Teach the elderly or persons with a disability how to communicate with their loved ones through email and Skype, and they instantly have a new friend. Computers can eliminate the barriers that many face when trying to communicate with people outside of their immediate community. One of my residents was able to use Skype to connect with her son who had been deployed for two years in the Middle East. It was a joyful moment and demonstrated the effectiveness of computers.

Facilitating programs and serving the residents is a good thing but strive to avoid co-dependency by your residents. You can be polite, personable and accessible without promising to be their savior. Use environmental and systematic approaches rather than relying heavily on individual clinical approaches. This allows residents to gain autonomy and a feeling of accomplishment. One example of this is when I noticed how one third of my residents had become dependent on the kindness of a local church meal program. I worked in partnership with the church and coordinated that the food distribution matched the residents' participation in our money management or eating smart meal program.

CHAPTER 8: YOUTH DEVELOPMENT AND FAMILY ENGAGEMENT

Make your youth programs measurable so that you can build on its success. One example is:

The participants of the DYM (Define Your Moment) program will experience a 10% improvement in their grade point average after six months of participation.

This book will provide RSCs assistances in identifying education performance indicators for each participant (as a means of objectively quantifying the results of a program, projects and services).

An RSC will become confident in setting goals such as: 90% of the DYM program participants will graduate from high school and will have a plan for life (higher education, military, employment, etc.) following high school graduation

Based on a student exit survey given twice a year, at least 90% of our DYM participants will indicate that they were made aware of topics in professional ethics, finances, goal setting, community service and nutrition.

Increasing the educational, social and economic strength of your residents:

How are you measuring the academic outcomes of your school age residents? Are your residents motivated about learning and their personal development? Do your residents have realistic, achievable goals? Are you providing opportunities for parents to be actively engaged in the educational, social, and physical development of their kids? R.A.C.E (Realizing Achievements through Continual Education) provides a platform that says yes to all four of these questions.

Goal: Residents will earn meters through personal development.

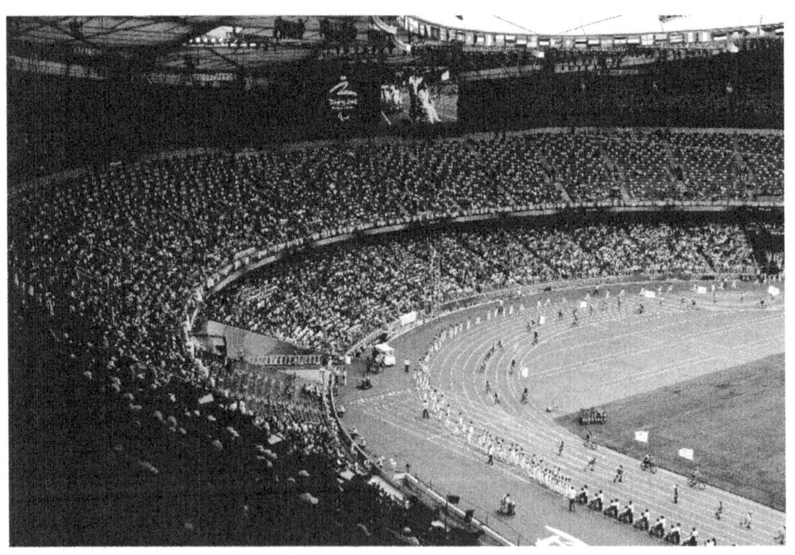

RACE will be updated weekly by the RSC

RSC will maintain a secure master sheet of the track

RSC will place the track poster in a highly visible location

In Orlando, Florida, Baltimore, Maryland and Richmond, Virginia, I was able to coordinate a program where adolescents engage in lifestyle development tasks to position themselves to win prizes. There are three levels to win under a track and field concept. Participant's names are listed at a starting line on the 4' wall picture shown above. Magnets are used to move participants along the track with the goal of crossing the finish line. There are three races: 100-meter dash, 4x100m relay and 1600m race. The first three participants to earn 100 meters win prizes: gold, silver and bronze for the 100-meter dash. Adolescents become excited seeing their name and progress in a highly visible public place. This fuels their ambition to do more of the Define Your Moment activities. I have used donated gifts as prizes including dinner for two at a three star restaurant, dress shirt, tie and cufflinks, designer sunglasses, dress shoes, two tickets to a local play, one-year gym membership and free dental teeth cleaning as prizes. These prizes are designed to promote cultural development. The 100-meter dash completion is designed to be achievable within two months, making it reachable without instant gratification. After building momentum for the program within the community, proceed to the 4x100m relay event. Now, you are teaching teamwork and participants are holding each other accountable to win. A team of four must each earn 100 meters to win. Again, go with three team winners: gold-silver-bronze. Place the winners on a podium and have a small ceremony with medals for the winning teams. Invite the parents to the ceremony for support. The 1600-meter race is designed to create longevity for the Define Your Moment program. It will take 4 to 5 months to reach the finish line for this race. The participants who stick with the program will become the face of your youth program, serving as ambassadors.

Define Your Moment by Earning Meters:

Read a book and write a 3 page report (book must be approved by RSC)	15
Submit a successful weekly progress report	3
Cook dinner for the household	3
Attend a BYE Study Hall	2
Participate in a BYE Community Service Project	8
Make the honor roll	25
Attend a BYE sponsored college tour	4
Take the PSAT, ACT or SAT (submit scores to RSC)	8
Complete and submit a college application	5

Pay rent on time	1
Parent/guardian participation in a BYE Community Service Project	6
Open a savings bank account ($25.00 minimum)	5
Complete the SAT question of the day (provide proof of the correct answer to the RSC)	1
Parent/guardian participation in PTA meetings	6
Participate in a DYM Workshop	5
Complete RSC and parental approved home chores	2

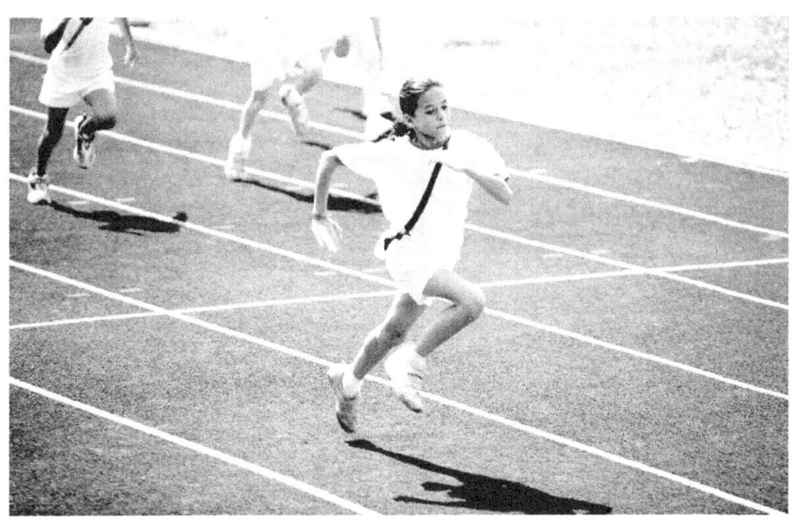

The Define Your Moment (DYM) workshops are where a lot of your growth, personal gains and development are going to occur. The RSC should facilitate weekly life skills workshops on subjects that best meet their population needs. Some suggested workshop topics include:

- the laws and dangers of sexting,

- the pros and cons of tattoos for adolescents,

- understanding credit scores and how to build credit,

- how to build a saving account for college,

- how to build a resume,

- bullying,

- conflict resolution,

- the art of networking,

- the effects of drug use,

- leadership development,

- how to participate in PTA meetings,

- the importance of goal setting,

- politics 101 – an introduction to policies,

- public speaking, etc.

Define Your Moment Weekly Progress Report:

Weekly progress reports are my favorite tool for monitoring the academic progress of student age residents. It allows you to track their level of engagement, enthusiasm for learning, relationship with teachers, connection with school and educational productivity. Teachers love this user-friendly tool because it gives them greater control over their students output and it promotes a partnership with the RSC for helping to advance the student's development. Students often embrace the weekly progress report after realizing significant gains in their learning and grade point average. Second, the submission of a weekly progress report is incentive based. I was able to establish a relationship with McDonalds and Subway, by which they agreed to provide free meals for students who submitted a successful weekly progress report. I would deliver as many as 30 value meals from McDonalds to deserving students in our after-school tutoring program or during their school lunch period for the submission of a successful weekly progress report. Students would converse amongst their peers about how committing to attending school and being productive can bring a tasty lunch. With Subway stores, I established a Football Player of the Week Program. Players who demonstrated extraordinary play on the football field and submitted a successful progress report for that week would receive lunch from the

Subway store. Under these terms, producing a successful progress report prevents students from earning "player of the week" solely based on their athletic performances. This reinforces the messages that education is important.

Sample Weekly Progress Report

RSC approved core courses only

DYM Participant Name: _______________________________

Date / Week of: _______________________________

Starting Blocks:

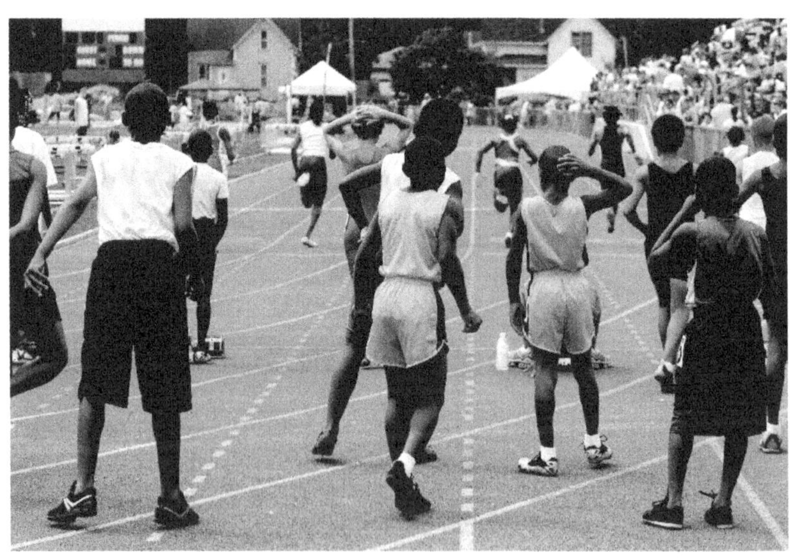

Subject:	Current With Homework	Class Absences	Class Participation	Class Behavior	Teacher's Initials	Comments:
Math	yes	1	high	very good, good	gf	Student is making progress
Biology	no	4	low			lacks interest
English	yes	1	moderate			uses text language in essays
History	no	1	high			performing at level
Spanish	yes	1	low			tutoring recommended

Education is the key ingredient to individual advancement, community building and greater access to resources and opportunities. Many high school students are dependent on their school's guidance counselor for career planning, college preparation, selecting a college and accessing funding for higher education. When you consider the United States average ratio (471 to 1) of students to guidance counselors, it becomes apparent that many students must take on career planning and college preparation tasks alone, with friends or under the influence of the media.

The American School Counselor Association recommends a ratio of 250 to 1 for guidance counselors to meet the individual needs of students adequately. The students to guidance counselor ratio in states where Beacon Communities operate are:

Connecticut	471 to 1
Maryland	357 to 1
Massachusetts	441 to 1
New York	392 to 1
Pennsylvania	377 to 1
Rhode Island	374 to 1
Virginia	315 to 1

In implementing the starting blocks program, your residents will have access to customized and individualized college preparation, career planning and life coaching services.

College preparation services should consist of:

- Locating scholarships
- SAT/ACT prep
- Completing college applications
- Writing winning essays
- Choosing the "right" college
- Navigating the college process
- Organizing college tours
- Career Planning:
- Career exploration / assessment
- Job search strategies
- Interviewing skills / practice
- Resume writing
- Life Coaching:
  1. balancing work and family
  2. career change, advancement, upward mobility
  3. adult education
  4. introduction to entrepreneurship

As we consider the schools that serve our communities, let's examine Blue Ridge Estates community in Richmond, Virginia:

1. Elizabeth Redd Elementary ranks 982nd out of 1001 Virginia elementary schools which directly serve their residents

2. Westover Hills Elementary ranks 810th out of 1001 Virginia elementary schools which directly serve their residents

3. Lucille Brown Middle ranks 236th out of 269 Virginia middle schools that directly serve Blue Ridge Estates residents.

4. George Wythe High ranks 246th out of 306 Virginia high schools that directly serve their residents.

In Richmond, 68% of Black males drop out of school. Let's not be completely dependent on schools to educate our kids; we must act. Nationally, 50% of people born into poverty will remain in a life of poverty. Fifty percent of Blacks males will be arrested by the age of 23. With knowledge of these statistics, wouldn't it be prudent to offer individual career planning and college preparation for residents in affordable housing. Make learning personal so that your residents have greater opportunities to grow and reach their full potentials. Companies such as Holmes Smith Consulting Service offer parents and adolescents opportunities for advancement by assessing their strengths, needs and equipping clients with the tools needed to achieve.

Often, when I ask residents to name what two products are most exported by the United States, I am met with a puzzled look. In fairness, this isn't a question often posed to most people. However, this question is relevant to residents who need assistance with career planning and college preparations. According to the United States Department of Commerce, agriculture is what the United States produces in abundance and exports throughout the world. Next is entertainment. Movies from the United States are seen throughout the world and United States athletes are beloved by many. Most residents are not interested in becoming farmers or manufacturers of mass foods. However, many residents are absolutely sold on the dream of being a movie star, a rap star, American idol winner and/or professional athlete. Perhaps this is why 66% of African American youths believe that athletics is their only way out of poverty and how they define success. Many colleges capitalize on the naïve dreams of our residents because colleges are aware that less than 1% of college athletes become professional athletes; 86% of college athletes live in poverty as they generate billions for the college and coaches. The average career lifespan in professional football is three years and 60% – 75% of professional football and basketball players file bankruptcy within three years of retiring. This is useful information in helping residents map out a realistic and sustainable career plan.

The DYM program will better equip our kids for competing in the arena of education. Failing schools typically share some characteristics: lower operating budget, low parental involvement, poor standardize test scores, unhealthy learning environment and high teacher turnover. The DYM program is a beginning to help our kids have a fighting chance at a quality education. Let's support our children's' educational needs. If you are unsure whether intervention is needed for residents of low socioeconomic communities, the Richmond Times Dispatch wrote the following article:

December 2013

<u>"teacher didn't walk away easily"</u>

"Conditions at school were deplorable.

"No soap, no toilet paper, mold growing on the walls.

"Educationally, it was a challenge to teach in a place where kids fought without consequences."

Martin Luther King Jr. Middle School posted a state worst 3% pass rate on seventh grade math assessments for 2011-2012 school years. The number jumped to 11 percent last year, still 59 points short of the state's minimum pass rate. This year (2013), the school is ranked last among 269 middle schools in the state. Sixty percent of what the U.S. exports is entertainment. So, is it any wonder that 66% of African American males believe that entertainment is their only means of success? What is the message that they are receiving from the media, and from society. 86% of college athletes live in poverty while the average division 1a football and basketball coach is a millionaire. As Resident Service Coordinators of family communities, do we ignore this information or do we adopt a plan to counteract the talent being lost from residents chasing the dream of being an entertainer.

I have done some research as to why some people fall by the way side, when others succeed. Why do some people fight for what they believe in and others don't? Why do some people define the moment while others let the moment define them? The answer is simple; those who achieve their goals tend to come from communities that are supportive and caring, with programs that are empowering, motivating and creates opportunities. A nurturing community is especially important for minorities in affordable housing communities. Some examples of achievements that have been made when higher learning institutions foundation is deeply rooted in nurturing and self-awareness are:

*Nine of the top ten colleges that graduate most of the African American students who go on to earn Ph.D.'s are Historical Black Colleges and Universities (HBCUs).

*More than 50 percent of the nation's African American public school teachers and 70 percent of African American dentists and physicians earned degrees at HBCUs.

*In 2000, Xavier University in New Orleans individually produced more successful African American medical school applications than John Hopkins, Harvard, and the University of Maryland combined. Two other HBCUs also placed in the top ten producers of medical school applicants include Morehouse and Spelman College.

*Almost half of the members of the Congressional Black Caucus attended an HBCU.

*Eight of the top nine producers of African American baccalaureates in mathematics were HBCUs: Morehouse College, South Carolina State University, Alabama State University, Spelman College, Southern University, Tennessee State University, Hampton University and Howard University

*Top producer of African American pharmacists is Florida A&M University.

HBCUs enroll upwards of 370,000 students and graduate a significant share of all African Americans receiving degrees. While comprising of only three percent of the nation's 3,688 institutions of higher learning, HBCUs mastered the art of delivering programs and hiring staff that inspires and supports students.

Howard University 2014 participated in a Mock trial team and advanced to the championship tournament. On March 22, 23, Howard competed against Princeton, Penn State, George Washington, Rutgers, American University and the University of Maryland.[3]

According to the Huffington Post, the young HBCU alums to watch in 2013 are:

Bomani Jones, Founder Old Soul Productions, LLC – Clark Atlanta University

Francena McCorory and Kellie Wells, United States Olympic Medalists, Hampton University

Craig Stokes, Creator Style Minute and My Vote Counts, - North Carolina A&T State University

---

[3] www.thinkhbcu.org

Aerial Ellis Partner, duGard Ellis Public Relations, - Tennessee State University

Colen Wiley, CEO Heygood Images Productions, - Hampton University

Nicholas M. Perkins, CEO Perkins Management Services Company Inc., - Fayetteville State University

Isaac Redman NFL Running Back, Pittsburg Steelers – Bowie State University

RSCs are a beacon of light for many of us, as we can't make it alone. (Dr. King was a man who realized that it is not how long you live but how well you live. And how well you live is defined by how productive you are with every single minute that God has blessed you with. Today is the day when we take back our kids, proclaim our destiny and become a people of pride – service – intelligence. If we fail to act, we will continue to see the rise of single parent households, the highest high school dropout rate, the highest incarceration rate, the highest incidence of preventable chronic illnesses, households with the lowest wealth and a people that have lost their way.

Harriet Tubman was a visionary who improved the lives of thousands. Who is today's Harriet Tubman? I think it could be you. The greatest riches on earth are obtained by those who use their time wisely. Many people forfeit their riches because they remain motionless when it's their season to go! Richness is forfeited by wasted time and untapped potential. The richest place on earth is not in the oil fields of Saudi Arabia, nor in the bank accounts of star athletes. Instead, the richest place is the graveyard, the prison and the street corner. In the graveyard, there are dreams that never became reality; records that were never broken, skills that were never used, talent that was never displayed and leadership that was never assumed. The graveyard is a place where billions of dollars' worth of potential is being buried every day, never to be seen or experienced again. To fulfill their destiny and to improve their lives, residents are at a greater advantage when a Resident Service Coordinator is partnering with them.

Therefore, it is important to encourage, motivate and inform your residents that the road to success is not straight. There is a curve called failure, a loop called confusion, speed bumps called friends, and traffic lights called peer pressure. But if residents have a spare tire called determination, an engine called perseverance, a support system called a

Resident Service Coordinator and a driver called their savior, they will make to a place called Success.[4]

Pass the Baton

Passing the baton is a proven mentorship program for high school students. Two high school upperclassmen will serve as mentors for a 9th and 10th grader within their respective community. Tasks include helping with study skills, building self-esteem, decision making and navigating the terrain of high school.

The two high school students in turn will be aligned with two mentors from the business community. This partnership will expose the high school upper classmen to professional careers, the culture of corporate America, adult responsibilities, setting goals, decision-making, the art of etiquette and financial planning.

The high school and parent(s) will be incorporated in the program to ensure that all parties are working on behalf of the students.

The RSC will monitor the interaction and relationships of the high school and business mentors.

---

[4] *The Artificial Rainbow*, Gregory Ford, 2013, www.artificialrainbow.com

This program is designed to help residents lead other residents to a place of success through self-empowerment.

The RSC will implement program evaluations and measurement tools to assess the program's effectiveness and the receptiveness of participants to the program.

The RSC will promote the program in the community to build on-going support.

Benefits of the DYM Program:

Residents will gain access to a wide range of support and opportunities needed to grow up healthy, caring and responsible.

Residents experience an increased sense of self-efficacy as they learn that they can influence real social challenges, problems and needs.

Residents experience higher academic achievement and interest in furthering their education.

Residents enhance their problem-solving skills, their abilities to work in teams, live in harmony as a community and planning abilities.

Residents experience an enhanced civic engagement attitude. Many leaders in public service speak about how they were nurtured, inspired and shaped in early experiences in community service or volunteering.

The DYM program cultivates connections between RSCs and the schools that our residents attend.

DYM can increase staff volunteer level of engagement, leadership capacity, and satisfaction with their work.

DYM will give residents an intentional strategy for addressing goals for learning and personal development through civic engagement and community service.

CHAPTER 9: INTERNSHIP

Many of the responsibilities of the Resident Service Coordinator coincide with the teaching of accredited social work programs. In light of this, it can be beneficial to the RSC to supervise a social work intern. If you do not have a social work degree, it is best to avoid supervising master level social work students.

Internship exposes the student to the functions of the social work profession and gives students the opportunity to apply classroom theories to real world problems. Affordable housing communities make for a learning environment because it exposures interns to the challenges people face in everyday living. You can only learn so much from reading books and listening to lectures even from the best instructors. Having a social work intern is beneficial to housing management organizations because this can be a training ground for maintaining a strong RSC workforce. According to the National Association of Colleges and Employers (NACE) 2009 survey, 35% of employer's fulltime, entry-level college hires came from their internship programs. If RSCs and property managers look at internships from a solution-based perspective, it's good news as well. Because, essentially, interns can help the RSC manage duties to accomplish the following immediate objectives:

Interns can help Resident Service Coordinators increase productivity. Setting up an internship program allows RSCs to take advantage of short-term support. The extra sets of hands help RSCs to be more productive, prevent them from becoming overburdened by side projects and free RSCs to handle more creative tasks where higher learning, strategic thinking is required.

Interns tend to bring novel perspectives, fresh ideas and specialized learning targeted at your population.

Affordable housing management organizations tend to be driven by the desire to help the most vulnerable population by providing quality housing coupled with life enhancing programs. Because of the needs complexity of residents, RSCs often rely on community alliances for support. Creating an internship program is an excellent way to give back to the community that supports your residents. Hosting internships not only helps students in your community get experience; it enhances the relationship between your organization and the academia community.

Through community partnerships, the community where I served as a Resident Service Coordinator was able to establish a comprehensive wellness program. The wellness clinic utilizes medical students, nursing students, pharmacy students and social work students to deliver preventative health care to a population plagued by chronic diseases, thanks to a well-organized internship program. By the end of year one, the wellness program served 108 residents out of a 247 resident community. The wellness program received national attention for its effectiveness to deliver critical service to the elderly and those with a disability, using a core of undergraduate and graduate student interns.

Note, when agreeing to take on an intern it is important to identify what outcomes the intern wishes to achieve.

I currently supervise an undergraduate student intern who works 24 hours a week at our location. I coordinate her task/assignments around her learning needs and the university social work curriculum. It is important to connect the various theories that are learned in class with real world experiences. Thus, Tiffany (my intern) has the opportunity to experience the practical implications of her learning. For example, as Tiffany takes social work research, we apply that to study issues such as hoarding in our community. With her human behavior course, I focus on planning programs or self-help groups to examine the external factors (environment, culture) and internal factors such as biological, social and psychological factors that influence our resident's behavior. With this knowledge, I am able to assign the intern to help facilitate programs such as Alcoholics Anonymous, the wellness clinic, adult learning and family advocacy. Having the intern complete the intake assessments is critical to teaching interviewing skills, identifying the strengths and needs of residents, developing an appropriate plan of care, reading non-verbal behavior, engaging a diversity of residents and quantifying information so that the RSC department can stay current with the needs of our ever-changing population.

Having an intern is beneficial but make sure their learning coincides with the RSC needs as well. Insure that the learning is measurable, challenging and rewarding. Each day, I sit down to discuss cases with the intern to explore how she would have handled the situation or to critique the manner in which she handled the situation. What I gain is an objective view of things from her and in addition, I am forced to be in tune with current literature around social work so that I operate alongside her with what is being taught in the classroom. And sometimes, I am able to realize my mistakes by reviewing material with her, and in this instance, having an intern is a win-win situation. There is additional paperwork, meetings and miscellaneous work that comes with the role of intern supervisor, so bear that in mind. The intern's professor often asks questions such as how has the student grown, what developmental needs does she need for the workforce, what ethical principles does the social work intern demonstrate, how has she influenced the policy development of Beacon? Provide documentation of the intern's people skills and what theories have he or she mastered in working with residents?

A psychology student intern might be suitable for the RSC program as well.

A student-learning plan might look like the following:

Learning Objectives

1. To gain knowledge about the transference and countertransference as it applies to client/student working relationships

2. To acquire professional case documentation skills and develop interviewing skills using motivational interviewing techniques and strategies

3. To gain experience with methods of client advocacy

4. To become proficient in facilitating groups and program development

5. To perform case management duties to contribute to policy development and be able to enforce policies in a professional manner

6. To establish goals and an individual plan of care for residents that meets their specific needs

7. To incorporate technology with the delivery of service to residents

8. To integrate theoretical learning to a practical setting

CHAPTER 10: IMPROVING RESIDENTS' PARTICIPATION

It is very frustrating to implement a great program and yet few residents participate. The time, energy and resources devoted to the program can make even the most seasoned RSC give up and throw in the towel. But before you do that, try this!

Host a brunch for your new residents from a certain year. Send out personalized invitations to your most recent move-ins and reminders to attend the brunch. The goal is to connect with your new residents, engage them, excite them and merge them into culture of the community. I hosted a new resident brunch by showing new residents a video of residents who have positive disposition, are actively engaged in RSC programs, who contribute to the community and who appreciate where they live. Showcasing existing residents gives new residents a lifeline to a potential friend. Following the video, I opened the doors of the community and brought in several residents to greet the new residents. Seasoned residents held signs such as "Ask me about Alcoholics Anonymous" – "Ask me about Connected Living" – "Ask me about the wellness clinic" and so forth. The residents used signs as a platform to share their story about how RSCs' programs have personally improved their quality of life. Testimonies from residents were genuine and gave other residents the courage to get involved. It has been proven that social programs promote better mental, physical and emotional health. Certain programs can aid in building trust and relationships so residents are comfortable coming to the Resident Service Coordinator.

The second plan that I am fond of using to increase participation in RSC programs is the Community Campaign. Similar to that of a blood drive, I posted thermal chart (like a thermometer) of various RSC programs. The bottom has the total number of residents within my community in red. Alongside each program's name is the apartment number of the residents who participate in that program. This offers a visual of what residents are interested in and it motivates residents who are isolated or uninvolved to participate in one of the programs to have their apartment represented on the chart. Like a donation chart or blood drive, there is a goal associated with the chart. My goal was to have 60% of the entire community engaged in one or more programs. It is critical to have residents utilizing services that your community is financially sponsoring.

The third plan is having a marketing strategy. Promote your programs using a marketing strategy, as this will help you define the goals of your residents and to develop programs to achieve them.

- Showcase the benefits of your RSC programs or services
- Have a budget to develop your marketing plan. No matter how small your community may be, effective marketing can increase residents' participation and the community morale.
- Creating and distributing flyers about programs is an effective tool. Flyers can keep you focused on engaging the residents. Also, consider how your residents access information about their community and discuss programs within the community.
- Have on-site public service announcements and contact the local media and small newspaper companies to shine light on your featured programs.

I began this chapter speaking about how frustrating low program participation can be. However, it is important that we be cognitive of the behavior that many of us demonstrate when it comes to asking for help. For instance, I can recall times when my peers would be struggling in their statistics class, yet wouldn't pursue tutorial assistance. There was a time when I had health issues and I agonized in pain daily. I would not access medical attention despite having medical insurance until my wife insisted I contact a physician. After receiving much needed medical care, I realized that I did not want to disrupt my lifestyle of being the provider and the track coach that was the reason for my not wanting to seek help. During times when traveled, I have even driven around for hours searching for a location, passing by countless gas stations where maps were sold and people were present to give directions. According to the psychology of help-seeking behavior, seeking assistance for one's situation is more complicated than people realize. So, instead of becoming frustrated that residents aren't utilizing a program or service despite the obvious benefits, try to be understanding and reflect on how you have struggled to accept assistance at some point in your life. There is a psychological cost to residents as they contemplate on whether to request assistance. Residents are evaluating whether the cost of seeking help outweighs the benefits of having it. My alcohol dependent residents might view the pains of withdrawal and the loss of a lifestyle as a greater cost than becoming sober and pursuing a path of healthier living.

For some, it is the value of freedom to make their own choice, even if it is a bad choice. Other residents might question your motive to help, thus making them resistant to accept the RSC assistance. Still others can feel that they would owe the Resident Service Coordinator something (and don't have the means to pay) if they participate in a program. To this, I communicate how much the residents' participation in these programs is rewarding to my professional and personal development. I also inform residents that their participation in programs or acceptance to service is an open invitation.

On the following page is an example of how a chart might look for a community of 249 residents. You could add a column for the Weekly Schedule to let your residents know when the program was available.

Program Names	Clients Participating
Eating Smart	22
Dental Care	45
I'm Okay	162
Wellness Clinic	110
Book Club	15
Connected Living	75
Spanish Class	2
Alcoholics Anonymous	2
Exercise Class	10
The People's Café	30
House Keeping	12
Money Talk	25
Dr. Transportation	25
Smoking Cessation	12
Art Class	10
Total Residents	**249**
Goal	60%
To Date*	144
Percentage Reached	**58%**

*Actual #of residents enrolled

Some residents participate in multiple programs

RSCs, we all have a limited time on earth. The big question is, how will you be remembered? Will you define the moment or let the moment define you? Defining your moment is about making the most of the time you have as a Resident Service Coordinator.

Made in United States
Orlando, FL
20 February 2023

30186986R00052